Timeless Radiance

Your Ultimate Guide to an Optimal Anti-Aging Regimen with Strategies for Glowing Skin, Vitality, and Graceful Aging

DR JOYCE A. MOORE

This book does not offer psychiatric or medical advice; it is just intended for informational and educational purposes. If you have specific concerns about your medical or mental health, please speak with a trained expert.

Copyright © 2024 by Dr Joyce A. Moore

amazon.com/author/joyceamoore

Introduction

Understanding the Aging Process

In a world where the pursuit of ageless beauty and vitality is a common aspiration, this comprehensive guide is your key to unlocking the secrets of a timeless and radiant existence. Aging is a natural part of life, but with the right knowledge and practices, you can enhance your well-being, embrace your journey, and age with grace.

In the following pages, we will dig into a handpicked array of science-backed methods, skincare regimens, and lifestyle choices meant to empower you in your search for young vitality. Whether you're just beginning your anti-aging journey or looking to fine-tune your existing regimen, "Timeless Radiance" offers insights that cater to all ages and stages of life.

Prepare to embark on a transformative experience as we explore the realms of skincare innovation, nutritional excellence, and holistic well-being. Let this guide be your companion on the path to radiant skin, boundless energy, and a renewed sense of confidence. Embrace the wisdom within these pages, and embark on a journey that goes beyond the surface – one that celebrates the beauty of aging while embracing the full spectrum of your timeless radiance.

Aging is a natural and inevitable aspect of the human experience, marking the continuous evolution and transformation of our bodies and minds. This intricate process encompasses a multitude of biological, psychological, and social changes, shaping the unique journey of each individual as they progress through the various stages of life.

Aging is a deep and complex process characterized by a symphony of biological, psychological, and social changes. While the process is unavoidable, the way an individual ages is impacted by a mix of genetic variables, lifestyle decisions, and the larger society environment. By understanding and embracing the multifaceted nature of aging, individuals can navigate this journey with resilience, wisdom, and a commitment to lifelong well-being. It is a journey that, when approached with mindfulness and purpose, can lead to a life of enduring significance and fulfillment.

Embracing the Journey

Now that we've uncovered some of the scientific aspects of aging, let's shift our focus to embracing the journey itself.

Aging is a natural part of life, and approaching it with a positive mindset can significantly impact how we experience the process.

1. Celebrating Life's Phases

Just as seasons change, our lives go through different phases. Each stage brings its own unique joys and experiences. We'll discuss how embracing these changes and appreciating the wisdom that comes with age can enrich our lives.

2. Redefining Beauty

In a world that often emphasizes youthful appearances, let's redefine what beauty means as we age. Beauty isn't confined to a specific age; it evolves and takes on new forms. We'll explore how embracing our changing appearance can lead to a more positive and confident self-image.

3. The Power of Mindset

Our thoughts shape our reality. Adopting a positive mindset towards aging can influence how we feel about ourselves and our overall well-being. We'll discuss practical strategies for cultivating a mindset that sees aging as an opportunity for growth and continued fulfillment.

4.   Building Meaningful Connections

Relationships are vital to our pleasure and well-being. Nurturing relationships with friends, family, and community becomes increasingly important as we get older. We'll look at how developing and maintaining meaningful connections leads to a more full and vibrant existence.

5. *Cultivating Self-Care Habits*

Self-care is a key element in embracing the aging process. We'll delve into simple yet effective self-care practices that promote physical, emotional, and mental well-being. These practices can enhance the quality of life and contribute to a positive aging experience.

Embracing the journey of aging is about more than just understanding the science; it's about appreciating the richness of life at every stage. This section aims to guide you in adopting a mindset that allows you to navigate the aging process with grace, finding joy, and fulfillment along the way. It's an invitation to celebrate the beauty of the evolving self and embrace the journey with open arms.

Chapter 1

The Science of Aging

Aging is a natural and complex process that unfolds within our bodies over time. In this chapter, we'll dive into the science behind aging, exploring the biological intricacies that contribute to this fascinating journey.

Unveiling the Biological Clock

In this section, we'll explore the basic science behind aging, breaking it down into simple terms to help you understand what's happening inside your body as time goes by.

1.1 The Cellular Basis of Aging:

Imagine your body is made up of tiny building blocks called cells. As we age, these cells go through changes. Some of them stop dividing and become what we call "senescent."It's as if they've retired from their typical work of proliferating and assisting our bodies in self-repair. We will investigate why this occurs and how it relates to the aging process

.1.2 *The Mitochondrial Connection:*

Think of mitochondria as tiny power plants within your cells. They generate energy to keep your body running smoothly. But over time, these power plants can get a bit worn out, producing "oxidative stress." We'll explore how this stress affects your cells and contributes to the aging journey.

1.3 *Environmental Factors and Aging:*

Now, consider that our bodies interact with the world around us. The air we breathe, the food we eat, and the sun we're exposed to can impact how we age. We'll talk about how our lifestyle choices and the environment influence the aging process, either speeding it up or slowing it down.

Genetic Factors and Aging

Next, let's look at how our genes, the instructions in our DNA, play a role in aging, for developing effective anti-aging strategies. In this section, we explore key aspects of the cellular basis of aging, shedding light on the processes that occur within individual cells as they navigate the journey of time.

2.1 The Genetics of Aging:

Genes are like your body's instruction manual. Some genes are connected to prolonged life, whereas others may accelerate the aging process. We will investigate these genetic elements and see how they affect how we age.

2.2 Epigenetics and Aging:

Epigenetics is like a volume control for genes. It can turn them up or down without changing the instructions. We'll see how lifestyle choices, like what we eat and how we manage stress, can adjust this volume and impact how our genes contribute to aging.
Knowing these basics will empower you to make choices that can positively influence how you age, supporting your journey toward timeless radiance.

The Biological Tapestry of Aging

Cellular Dynamics

Aging begins at the microscopic level, within the trillions of cells that compose our bodies. Over time, cells undergo a phenomenon known as cellular senescence, a state where they cease to divide. This reduction in cell replication contributes to the gradual decline in tissue regeneration and repair, a hallmark of aging.

Telomeres and Genetic Clocks:

Chromosomes, which house our genetic material, are capped by protective structures called telomeres. With each cell division, telomeres shorten, acting as a biological clock that tracks cellular aging. This process is intricately linked to the lifespan of cells and contributes to the overall aging of the organism.

Mitochondrial Health:

Within our cells, mitochondria serve as energy powerhouses, converting nutrients into usable energy. The wear and tear on these vital structures over time can lead to oxidative stress, impacting cellular function and accelerating the aging process.

Genetic Factors:

Our genetic makeup significantly influences how we age. Certain genes are associated with increased longevity, while others may predispose individuals to age-related conditions. The interplay between inherited genetic factors and environmental influences creates a complex mosaic of aging experiences.

The Environmental Symphony

Lifestyle Impact:

Choices we make in our daily lives, from diet and exercise to sleep and stress management, play a pivotal role in how we age. Healthy lifestyle habits can mitigate the impact of aging, promoting overall well-being and vitality.

Environmental Exposures:

The world around us, with its pollutants, radiation, and other environmental factors, contributes to the aging process. Understanding and reducing our exposure to hazardous materials helps slow the aging process.

The Psychological Landscape

Cognitive Aging:

Mental processes undergo changes with age, influencing memory, processing speed, and cognitive flexibility. While some decline is natural, engaging in intellectually stimulating activities can help maintain cognitive function.

Emotional Well-being:

Aging often brings with it a wealth of experiences and wisdom, contributing to emotional resilience. However, challenges such as loss and transition can impact mental health. Cultivating social connections and seeking support are crucial elements in maintaining emotional well-being.

Genetic Factors and Aging

Unraveling the Code of Time

Genetic factors play a pivotal role in the aging process, shaping the trajectory of an individual's journey through the various stages of life. The intricate dance between inherited genes and the environment contributes to the diversity of aging experiences among individuals. Let's explore the fascinating world of genetic factors and aging.

1. The Genetic Blueprint:

At the core of genetic factors in aging is the information encoded in our DNA, the intricate blueprint that dictates the formation and functioning of every cell in our bodies. The genome, comprised of genes, provides instructions for processes crucial to our development, health, and longevity.

2. Longevity Genes:

Some individuals are endowed with what scientists call "longevity genes." These genes, which are frequently connected with a long lifespan, help promote cellular repair, withstand stress, and preserve general health. Studying these genes sheds light on the underlying factors that lead to a longer and better life.

3. Accelerated Aging Genes:

Conversely, certain genetic variations may predispose individuals to accelerated aging. These genes can impact critical cellular functions, leading to increased vulnerability to age-related diseases and a faster decline in overall health. Understanding these genetic factors is crucial for identifying potential risk factors and developing targeted interventions.

4. Telomeres and Aging:

Telomeres, the protective caps at the ends of chromosomes, serve as a molecular clock that influences the aging process. The activity of the enzyme telomerase, which helps maintain the length of telomeres, is influenced by genetic factors. Variations in genes associated with telomerase can affect cellular aging and, consequently, impact overall longevity.

5. Epigenetics:

The study of epigenetics adds a layer of complexity to the genetic narrative. Epigenetic modifications are changes in gene activity that do not involve alterations to the underlying DNA sequence. Environmental factors and lifestyle choices can influence epigenetic patterns, affecting how genes are expressed and contributing to the aging process.

6. Genetic Diversity and Aging:

The mosaic of genetic diversity across populations contributes to the wide spectrum of aging experiences. While genetics plays a significant role, it interacts with various environmental factors, creating a nuanced interplay that defines how individuals age. By understanding this complexity allows for a more personalized approach to health and wellness in the aging population.

7. Genetic Research and Anti-Aging Strategies:

Advances in genetic research hold promise for developing targeted anti-aging interventions. Scientists explore ways to manipulate genes or mimic the effects of longevity genes to promote healthier aging. Personalized medicine, tailored to an individual's genetic profile, is on the horizon, offering the potential for more effective and precise approaches to aging-related conditions.

8. Ethical Considerations:

As the field of genetic research progresses, ethical considerations become paramount. Balancing the potential benefits of genetic interventions with concerns related to privacy, equity, and unintended consequences is crucial in shaping the future of genetic-based anti-aging strategies.

In essence, genetic factors are a fundamental part of the aging narrative, influencing how our bodies respond to the passage of time. While some aspects of our genetic makeup are beyond our control, understanding the role of genetics in aging empowers individuals to make informed lifestyle choices and engage in proactive health measures that can positively impact the aging process. As science continues to unravel the complexities of our genetic code, the potential for personalized, genetically informed approaches to aging holds promise for a future where individuals can age with resilience, vitality, and grace.

Chapter 2

Skincare Essentials

As the sands of time continue to shape our journey, the care we extend to our skin becomes a testament to our commitment to graceful aging. Discover the key elements of a skincare regimen designed to enhance the radiance of aging skin, embracing the wisdom that comes with time.

Building a Solid Skincare Routine

Skincare is not just about beauty; it's a commitment to the health and vitality of your skin. In this chapter, we'll delve into the essential elements of a robust skincare routine that will leave your skin feeling refreshed, radiant, and well-nourished.

1.1 Understanding the Basics

Skincare is a journey, and the first step is to understand your skin type and its unique needs. We'll explore the foundational elements of a skincare routine, from cleansing to moisturizing, setting the stage for a comprehensive approach to your daily regimen.

1.2 The Importance of Consistency

Consistency is essential in skincare. We'll talk about how important it is to set and keep to a routine in order to provide your skin with regular and balanced treatment.

Choosing the Right Products for Your Skin Type

Understanding your skin's individual characteristics is crucial for selecting products that cater to its specific needs. This section will guide you through the process of identifying your skin type and choosing the right products accordingly.

2.1 Skin Typing: Decoding Your Unique Needs

Discover whether your skin is oily, dry, combination, or sensitive. We'll provide insights into recognizing the signs and understanding the characteristics of each skin type, empowering you to make informed choices for your skincare arsenal.

2.2 Tailoring Products to Your Skin's Needs

Not all skincare products are created equal. Learn how to select cleansers, moisturizers, and other essentials that align with your skin type. We'll explore the world of ingredient labels, demystifying the key components that contribute to effective skincare.

3. Incorporating Serums and Actives

Serums and active ingredients are the powerhouse of any skincare routine, offering targeted solutions to specific concerns. This section will guide you through the integration of serums and active ingredients into your daily regimen.

3.1 The Role of Serums in Skincare

Understand the benefits of serums and how they can address specific skin concerns such as hydration, anti-aging, and brightening. We'll explore the different types of serums available and how to incorporate them seamlessly into your routine.

3.2 Navigating Actives:

A Guide to Potency

Actives, including ingredients like retinol, vitamin C, and hyaluronic acid, can transform your skincare routine. Learn how to navigate the potency of these ingredients, ensuring their optimal efficacy while avoiding potential pitfalls.

We need to have a thorough grasp of the principles of skincare, how to address your skin's specific demands, and the transformational potential of serums and actives. Begin your journey to bright and healthy skin as we explore the world of skincare basics together.

Chapter 3

Nutritional Foundations for Youthful Living

In the pursuit of timeless vitality, the importance of nourishment cannot be overstated. "Nutritional Foundations for Youthful Living" is a chapter dedicated to unlocking the potential of wholesome nutrition in promoting radiant skin and fostering an ageless lifestyle. Join us as we explore the role of antioxidants, the superfoods that can transform your skin from within, and the profound impact of hydration on the aging process.

1. The Role of Antioxidants in Anti-Aging:

Discover the extraordinary power of antioxidants in combating the effects of time on your skin. This section delves into the science behind antioxidants, understanding how they neutralize free radicals, reduce oxidative stress, and contribute to a vibrant and youthful complexion. Uncover the key sources of antioxidants and learn how to incorporate them into your daily diet for maximum anti-aging benefits.

2. Superfoods for Radiant Skin:

Supercharge your skincare journey by embracing the incredible potential of superfoods. From nutrient-rich berries to omega-3 fatty acid-packed fish, we explore a curated selection of foods that offer unparalleled benefits for promoting radiant and healthy skin. Learn how these superfoods can enhance your overall well-being and contribute to a luminous complexion that defies the passage of time.

3. Hydration and Its Impact on Aging:

Water, the elixir of life, takes center stage in this section as we uncover its transformative impact on the aging process. Explore the crucial role of hydration in maintaining skin elasticity, promoting cellular function, and preventing premature aging. Dive into practical tips on staying adequately hydrated and integrating hydrating foods into your diet for a comprehensive approach to youthful living.

Nutritional Foundations for Youthful Living is an exploration of the symbiotic relationship between what we consume and the radiance we project. As we navigate the realms of antioxidants, superfoods, and hydration, we invite you to embrace a holistic approach to nourishment that not only fuels your body but also becomes an essential element in your anti-aging arsenal. Join us on this journey towards a lifestyle that nourishes not just your skin but your entire sense of well-being.

Chapter 4

1. The Mind-Body Connection:

1.1 Understanding the Mind-Body Link:

Explore the intricate relationship between mental and physical well-being. Delve into the ways in which thoughts and emotions influence overall vitality, unraveling the scientific foundations of the mind-body connection and its impact on the aging process.

1.2 Learn practical ways for cultivating mindfulness and awareness in daily life:
Learn how to balance your mental and physical well-being using meditation techniques and mindful breathing exercises. Explore the

skill of living in the present moment and its potential to improve overall life pleasure.

2. Stress Management Techniques:

2.1 Unraveling the Impact of Stress:

Delve into the effects of stress on the body and mind, understanding its potential to accelerate the aging process. Gain insights into the physiological responses to stress and how chronic stress can contribute to various health issues. Recognize the importance of managing stress for a holistic approach to well-being.

2.2 Practical Stress Reduction Strategies:

Explore a toolkit of practical stress management techniques designed to restore balance and tranquility. From mindfulness practices and progressive muscle relaxation to time management strategies, discover approaches that align with your lifestyle. Learn how to create a serene mental landscape amidst life's challenges.

3. Incorporating Exercise for Longevity:

3.1 The Fountain of Youth in Physical Activity:

Uncover the transformative effects of exercise on the aging process. Delve into the science behind how regular physical activity positively influences not only physical health but also cognitive function and emotional well-being. Understand the role of exercise as a potent tool for promoting longevity.

3.2 Tailoring Exercise to Your Lifestyle:

Embark on a personalized fitness journey by exploring various forms of exercise suited to your preferences and abilities. Find the ideal mix that fits your lifestyle, from aerobic exercises and strength training to contemplative movement techniques such as yoga. Discover how to make exercise a fun and sustainable part of your everyday routine.

4. Navigating the Social Realm Interpersonal Relationships:

The quality of relationships becomes increasingly vital as we age. Building and maintaining social connections contribute not only to emotional well-being but also to physical health.

4.1 Societal Perceptions:

Societal attitudes toward aging can influence individual experiences.

Embracing a positive perspective on aging challenges stereotypes and fosters a culture that values the contributions of individuals at every stage of life. Strategies for Graceful

4.2 Aging Holistic Health Approach:

Embracing a comprehensive approach that considers physical, mental, and emotional well-being is essential for graceful aging. This involves eating a well-balanced diet, exercising regularly, and prioritizing mental and emotional wellness.

4.3 Continued Learning and Engagement:

Staying intellectually active through lifelong learning and pursuing hobbies fosters cognitive vitality. Engaging in meaningful activities contributes to a sense of purpose and fulfillment.

4.4 Adaptability and Resilience:

Aging often involves adapting to changing circumstances. Developing resilience and a flexible mindset helps individuals navigate life's challenges with grace and optimism.

Dive deep into understanding the mind-body connection, unraveling the intricate dance that defines how our mental state influences our overall health. Delve into the scientific foundations that underscore the profound impact our thoughts and emotions have on the aging process, unveiling the interconnected realms that shape our well-being.

Chapter 5

Lifestyle Habits for Ageless Living

In the pursuit of ageless living, adopting healthy lifestyle habits is paramount. This chapter delves into practices that contribute to a vibrant and enduring life, focusing on the rejuvenating power of quality sleep, the protective benefits of sun care, and the transformative effects of quitting harmful habits.

1. Quality Sleep for Skin Renewal:

1.1 Unlocking the Secrets of Beauty Sleep:

Quality sleep is a cornerstone of ageless living, offering a time for the body to repair and renew itself. Dive into the science of sleep and its profound impact on skin health. Explore the stages of sleep that facilitate cellular repair, collagen production, and the reduction of inflammation, contributing to a radiant and youthful complexion.

1.2 Practical tips for restorative sleep:

Discover practical ways to improve the quality of your sleep. Learn how to optimize your sleep for optimum skin renewal, from developing a regular sleep schedule to creating a peaceful sleeping environment. Discover the comprehensive advantages of adequate sleep, which go beyond skin health to total well-being.

2. Sun Protection and Its Anti-Aging Benefits:

2.1 The Sun's Dual Nature: Friend and Foe

While the sun is a source of vitality, excessive exposure can accelerate aging. Understand the dual nature of sunlight and its impact on skin aging. Delve into the science of UV radiation, free radicals, and how they contribute to wrinkles, fine lines, and other signs of premature aging.

2.2 Empowering Your Skin with Sun Care:

Explore the essential role of sun protection in maintaining youthful skin. From broad-spectrum sunscreen to protective clothing, learn how to shield your skin from harmful UV rays. Uncover the anti-aging benefits of diligent sun care, preventing sun damage and preserving your skin's elasticity and radiance over time.

3. Quitting harmful habits:

3.1 Breaking Free from Aging Accelerators

Harmful habits, such as smoking and excessive alcohol consumption, can expedite the aging process. Examine the impact of these habits on skin health and overall well-being. Understand how smoking accelerates collagen breakdown, leading to premature wrinkles, while excessive alcohol intake dehydrates the skin, contributing to a lackluster complexion.

3.2 The Liberation of Healthy Choices:

Empower yourself to break free from harmful habits and embrace a lifestyle that promotes ageless living. Discover the transformative effects of quitting smoking and moderating alcohol intake on skin rejuvenation. Embrace the liberation of healthy choices, paving the way for a future marked by vitality, resilience, and timeless beauty.

Incorporating these lifestyle habits into your daily routine opens the door to ageless living, empowering you to nurture your skin, protect it from external stressors, and make choices that contribute to a resilient and vibrant life.

Chapter 6

Advanced Anti-Aging Techniques

In the ever-evolving landscape of skincare, the pursuit of ageless beauty has ushered in a new era of advanced anti-aging techniques. This chapter serves as a gateway to the forefront of innovation, exploring transformative methodologies that transcend traditional skincare practices.

1. Exploring Retinoids and Peptides:

1.1 Unveiling the Power of Retinoids:

Retinoids, derived from vitamin A, stand as stalwart soldiers in the war against aging. Delving deep into the science, we uncover their ability to stimulate collagen production, accelerate cell turnover, and minimize the appearance of fine lines and wrinkles. From over-the-counter options to prescription formulations, we navigate the spectrum of retinoids and unravel the intricacies of incorporating them into your skincare arsenal.

1.2 Peptides: The Building Blocks of Youthful Skin:

In the realm of molecular magic, peptides emerge as the unsung heroes. Serving as the building blocks of proteins, peptides play a pivotal role in maintaining skin elasticity and firmness. Here, we explore the science behind peptides, understanding their contribution to collagen synthesis and their transformative effects on the overall texture and resilience of the skin. Peer into the world of peptide-infused products and unlock the potential of these microscopic marvels.

2. Non-Invasive Cosmetic Procedures:

2.1 A Gentle Approach to Rejuvenation:

The era of non-invasive cosmetic procedures has dawned, offering rejuvenation without the need for surgical intervention. Navigate the landscape of dermal fillers, Botox, and laser therapies. Understand how these minimally invasive techniques delicately address specific aging concerns, providing a nuanced and refined approach to achieving youthful aesthetics. Explore the advantages, considerations, and the artistry involved in these procedures.

2.2 The Art of Facial Rejuvenation:

Facial rejuvenation becomes an art form as we delve into techniques that harmonize with your unique features. From addressing wrinkles to combating sagging skin, explore the precision and artistry of non-invasive procedures. Gain insights into the consultation process, personalized treatment plans, and the role of skilled practitioners in achieving natural-looking results. Uncover the secrets of facial rejuvenation without compromising the essence of your individuality.

3. Cutting-Edge Innovations in Skincare:

3.1 The Science of Skincare Advancements:

Step into the future with a glimpse into the latest scientific advancements in skincare. From personalized formulations based on individual genetic profiles to the integration of artificial intelligence in skincare diagnostics, we explore the cutting-edge technologies shaping the next frontier of anti-aging. Understand how these innovations redefine the possibilities of personalized and effective skincare regimens.

3.2 Futuristic Trends in Anti-Aging:

Embark on a journey into the future of anti-aging with emerging technologies and trends. Peer into the realms of stem cell therapy, nanotechnology, and gene editing. Explore how these futuristic approaches hold the potential to revolutionize skincare, pushing the boundaries of age-defying interventions. Uncover the promises, ethical considerations, and the transformative possibilities that lie on the horizon.

This chapter transcends the ordinary, offering a glimpse into the realm where science meets artistry, where innovation fuses with tradition. As you explore retinoids, peptides, non-invasive procedures, and cutting-edge innovations, you embark on a journey that goes beyond conventional boundaries, embracing the transformative power of advanced anti-aging techniques.

Chapter 7

Tailoring Your Regimen to Your Age

In the pursuit of ageless beauty, understanding the nuances of skincare at different stages of life is essential. This chapter delves into the intricacies of tailoring your skincare regimen to your age, offering anti-aging strategies for every life stage and insights into adjusting your routine as you gracefully journey through the years.

1. Anti-Aging Strategies for Every Life Stage:

1.1 Embracing Youthful Radiance - 20s and 30s:

Explore preventive measures and early interventions to maintain youthful skin in your 20s and 30s. From establishing a solid foundation with sunscreen to incorporating antioxidants, learn how to safeguard your skin and lay the groundwork for a resilient complexion. Understand the importance of hydration and the early signs of aging to address them proactively.

1.2 Navigating the Transition - 40s and 50s:

As your skin undergoes changes in your 40s and 50s, discover strategies to navigate this transitional phase. Explore the role of collagen-boosting ingredients, such as retinoids and peptides, in combating fine lines and loss of elasticity. Tailor your routine to address specific concerns like hyperpigmentation and explore advanced anti-aging techniques that align with the evolving needs of your skin.

1.3 Embracing Graceful Aging - 60s and Beyond:

In your 60s and beyond, embrace the beauty that comes with age and adapt your skincare routine accordingly. Explore nourishing formulations that prioritize hydration and skin barrier support. Understand the importance of gentle exfoliation and continued sun protection. Embrace a holistic approach that fosters well-being while maintaining the health and vitality of your skin.

2. Adjusting Your Routine as You Age:

2.1 Adapting to Changing Needs:

Your skin's needs evolve over time, and adapting your routine is key to effective skincare. Explore how to modify your regimen in response to changes in skin texture, elasticity, and resilience. Understand the impact of hormonal shifts and environmental factors, and tailor your routine to address specific challenges associated with aging.

2.2 Holistic Wellness Integration:

Aging gracefully involves more than skincare; it encompasses holistic well-being. Learn to integrate lifestyle habits, including nutrition, exercise, and stress management, into your routine. Understand the symbiotic relationship between mental and physical well-being and how it contributes to a radiant and ageless presence.

This is a thorough handbook that provides specific solutions for each stage of life and practical advice on how to change your skincare routine as you age. As you manage the transitions and appreciate the beauty of each life stage, arm yourself with information that is relevant to the changing demands of your skin and well-being.

Chapter 8

Embracing Graceful Aging

As we embark on the journey of embracing graceful aging, this chapter invites you to explore the profound beauty that emanates from wisdom, experience, and the nurturing of self-love and confidence. Through introspection and intentional practices, discover how the passage of time becomes a canvas for personal growth and an affirmation of your unique, evolving beauty.

1. The Beauty of Wisdom and Experience:

1.1 A Canvas Painted by Time:

Delve into the beauty that emerges from a life rich in experiences and wisdom.

Understand how the passage of time shapes not only the external features but also the internal landscape of one's character. Explore the concept of beauty evolving with age and the empowerment that comes from embracing the unique story etched onto your being.

1.2 Wisdom-Infused Radiance:

Wisdom is a timeless beacon that illuminates one's presence. Explore the radiant qualities that wisdom imparts to your aura and how a depth of understanding enhances your overall allure. Acknowledge the value of life lessons, resilience, and the continuous journey towards self-discovery in cultivating an enduring and captivating presence.

2. Cultivating Self-Love and Confidence:

2.1 The Art of Self-Love:

Explore the art of self-love as a key component of graceful aging. Understand how accepting oneself, warts and all, leads to a radiant and confident personality. Investigate techniques that promote self-compassion, acceptance, and enjoyment of the unique beauty that comes with each passing year.

2.2 Confidence as a Timeless Elegance:

Confidence is the truest adornment, enhancing one's allure regardless of age. Uncover the transformative power of confidence and how it complements the physical aspects of aging. Embrace exercises in self-assurance, from positive affirmations to setting and achieving personal goals, fostering an enduring sense of confidence that radiates from within.

2.3 Navigating Societal Beauty Standards:

Address the societal narratives around aging and beauty standards. Explore strategies to navigate societal expectations while staying true to your authentic self. Embrace the liberation that comes from breaking free from stereotypical norms, allowing your unique beauty to shine irrespective of societal dictates.

3. *Harmony of Inner and Outer Beauty:*

3.1 Holistic Wellness for Aging Gracefully:

Aging gracefully involves a harmonious blend of inner and outer well-being. Explore practices that prioritize mental, emotional, and physical health. From nurturing meaningful relationships to engaging in activities that bring joy, understand how holistic wellness contributes to a radiant and ageless presence.

3.2 The Elegance of a Life Well-Lived:

Reflect on the elegance that emanates from a life well-lived. Celebrate accomplishments, cultivate gratitude, and embrace the richness of your journey. Explore how an authentic and purposeful life adds a timeless allure to your overall presence, creating a narrative of elegance and fulfillment.

In this chapter, the journey of embracing graceful aging unfolds as a celebration of wisdom, experience, self-love, and confidence As you traverse the complexities of inner and outer beauty, may you find inspiration in the beauty that endures and radiates from the depths of a life well lived.

Chapter 9

Japanese Wisdom for Longevity

In the quest for a vibrant and enduring life, the Japanese people have long been revered for their longevity and holistic approach to well-being.

This chapter unravels the cultural tapestry of Japan, exploring the lifestyle choices, dietary habits, and mindset that contribute to their exceptional health and longevity.

1. Embracing the Okinawan Way of Life:

1.1 Nourishment from Nature:

Venture into Okinawa, often referred to as the "Island of Longevity." Explore the Okinawan diet, rich in plant-based foods, sweet potatoes, and green tea. Understand how the Okinawan people prioritize nutrient-dense, locally sourced ingredients that form the foundation of their longevity-promoting meals.

1.2 Hara Hachi Bu - The Art of Mindful Eating:

Delve into the practice of "Hara Hachi Bu," an Okinawan mantra encouraging mindful eating. Uncover the wisdom of stopping eating when one is 80% full, fostering a balanced relationship with food and preventing overconsumption. Learn how this simple practice contributes to weight management and overall well-being.

2. Ikigai: Finding Purpose in Life:

2.1 The Essence of Ikigai:

Explore the concept of "Ikigai," a unique amalgamation of passion, vocation, mission, and profession that gives life meaning. Understand how the pursuit of purpose and fulfillment contributes to a sense of contentment and longevity among the Japanese people.

2.2 Engaging in Lifelong Learning:

Witness the commitment to lifelong learning as a cornerstone of Japanese longevity. From traditional arts to contemporary skills, discover how the Japanese embrace continuous learning, stimulating their minds and fostering a sense of curiosity throughout their lives.

3. Holistic Well-Being: Mind, Body, and Spirit:

3.1 Balancing Stress through Mindfulness: Uncover the Japanese approach to stress management through mindfulness practices such as meditation, tea ceremonies, and nature appreciation. Investigate how these routines help to a peaceful and focused frame of mind, lowering stress and enhancing mental health.

3.2 The Role of Physical Activity:

Embark on a journey into the Japanese commitment to physical activity. From daily walks to traditional martial arts practices like Tai Chi, discover how incorporating movement into daily life contributes to physical health, flexibility, and longevity.

4. Community and Social Connections:

4.1 The Importance of Social Bonds:
Understand the significance of close-knit communities in Japanese culture. Explore how strong social bonds, regular social interactions, and a sense of belonging contribute to mental health, emotional well-being, and longevity.

4.2 Ageing with Dignity:

Witness the respect and care afforded to the elderly in Japanese society. Explore the concept of "Respect for the Aged Day" and the cultural emphasis on intergenerational connections, showcasing how aging is viewed with reverence and dignity.

As we delve into the intricacies of Japanese wisdom for longevity, this chapter serves as an invitation to adopt elements of their lifestyle—nourishing not just the body but also the mind and spirit. Embrace a thoughtful lifestyle, discover your Ikigai, and be inspired by Japan's holistic approach to well-being for a life of energy and longevity.

Conclusion

Your Personalized Journey to Timeless Radiance

As we bring this transformative odyssey to a close, it is not merely the end of a book but the commencement of a chapter in your personalized journey towards timeless radiance. Throughout these pages, we've ventured into the realms of science, self-care, and the profound beauty that accompanies each stage of life.

Your beauty, like the universe, is in constant expansion—ever-evolving, ever-becoming. The wisdom shared here is not a prescription but a compass, guiding you through the vast terrain of self-discovery. It's an invitation to explore the intricate balance between science and intuition, the external and internal, the ephemeral and enduring.

Remember, beauty is not a static destination; it's a dynamic, personalized journey. Your skin tells a story, etched with the imprints of laughter, resilience, and the gentle touch of time. Embrace the wrinkles as chapters of joy, the fine lines as whispers of wisdom, and the evolving contours as a testament to the ceaseless dance between past, present, and future.

In these pages, you've explored the alchemy of skincare rituals, harnessed the power of advanced anti-aging techniques, and learned to adapt your regimen to the unique tapestry of your age. Beyond the serums and treatments lies the essence of embracing graceful aging—cultivating self-love, confidence, and a harmonious balance between inner and outer well-being.

Now, as you stand at the precipice of your personalized journey to timeless radiance, recognize the beauty that resides within the crevices of your uniqueness. Let the wisdom gathered here be the fuel that propels you forward, and let your personalized skincare routine be a sacred ritual of self-care—a homage to the magnificent canvas of your being.

The mirror reflects more than just physical characteristics; it catches the spirit of a fulfilling life. Your eternal glow is not an attempt at unreachable perfection, but rather a celebration of honesty, perseverance, and the magnificent beauty that exudes from your very core.

So, go forth with confidence, embrace each chapter of your life, and let the glow of timeless radiance be an eternal flame that illuminates your path. This is not just a conclusion; it's a commencement—an invitation to live, love, and glow with the luminosity of your own unique brilliance. May your journey be radiant, your spirit be ageless, and your beauty be a testament to the timeless grace within you.

www.ingramcontent.com/pod-product-compliance
Lightning Source LLC
Chambersburg PA
CBHW031328250726
48656CB00005B/2028